UNFORGETTABLE
JOURNEY

UNFORGETTABLE JOURNEY

Tips to Survive Your Parent's Alzheimer's Disease

Anne P. Hill

iUniverse, Inc.
New York   Bloomington

Unforgettable Journey
Tips to Survive Your Parent's Alzheimer's Disease
Second Edition

iUniverse books may be ordered through booksellers or by contacting:

iUniverse
1663 Liberty Drive
Bloomington, IN 47403
www.iuniverse.com
1-800-Authors (1-800-288-4677)

Because of the dynamic nature of the Internet, any Web addresses or links contained in this book may have changed since publication and may no longer be valid. The views expressed in this work are solely those of the author and do not necessarily reflect the views of the publisher, and the publisher hereby disclaims any responsibility for them.

ISBN: 978-1-4502-4176-2 (pbk)
ISBN: 978-1-4502-4177-9 (ebk)

Printed in the United States of America

iUniverse rev. date: 7/23/10

Contents

Acknowledgments

Thank you, Dr. Marian Hodges, for being my mother's doctor and for reading early drafts of this book. You are the best. Thank you, Dr. Shirin Sukumar, for your friendship and advice, your thoughtful comments on this book, and for my goddaughter! Thank you, Dr. Kevin Smith, for your years of experience, your compassion, your support for this book, and, in this day and age, for making house calls! Thank you, Margaret Murphy Carley, for the best—and most concise—advice ever given to anyone with a parent with Alzheimer's disease. Thank you to many years of caregivers who have taught me so much: Nisha, Lulan, Tedi, Daleen, Sandy, and Andrew among others. Thank you, Linda Landon, for all your support and encouragement.

Thank you, Sara Zwinger Roberts, for hours and hours of editing and suggestions. Thank you, Jane Zwinger, for your thoughtful illustrations that captured my heart and which my mother would have loved had she been able to see them. Thank you to the many other friends who read and commented as I wrote this book: Evan and Dillon Henry and the rest of the Henry clan, Dr. Mark and Colleen

O'Hollaren, Dr. Jim and Karin Chesnutt, Donna Proffit, Shauna Krieger, and others.

Thank you Betty Trowbridge and the prayer team at Multnomah Presbyterian Church for praying me through Mom's illness.

Thank you to the residents, some past and some present, of the memory care residence where Mom lives, from whom I have learned so much and whom I have come to love. You have brightened my life.

Last, and most important, thank you to my husband, Jeff, and our sons, Chet and Andy, for abiding with me on this long, long journey of Mom's illness.

Foreword

Alzheimer's disease is one of the fastest-growing problems facing our nation and its aging population. When a parent develops Alzheimer's disease, everything changes. This change becomes dramatic, often in a brief period of time. Adult children encounter new responsibilities at what may be the busiest time of their lives. The role reversal that develops can feel uncomfortable and awkward; unfortunately, there are no "playbooks" for how family members are to navigate their new roles. The burdens on families occur at a time when adult children are facing their own demands and responsibilities (children and careers, for example). Information may be needed quickly, but they have very little time in their lives to devote to learning. The burden can become overwhelming.

This book will help. Anne's experience with her mother is typical of the challenges of having a parent with Alzheimer's disease. Her approach, ideas, and solutions will be helpful to adult children as they learn to help their parent navigate the complexities of Alzheimer's disease.

There are many books written about Alzheimer's disease. The concise nature and easy readability of this book will make it an effective tool for family members with a parent who has dementia. The upbeat nature and "Tips" section at the end of each chapter helps the book read in much the same way that a supportive conversation with a friend would be to the reader. I heartily recommend this book to the adult children of my patients with Alzheimer's disease.

Kevin R. Smith, MD
Assistant Professor of Psychiatry
Director, Geriatric Psychiatry Clinic
Oregon Health & Sciences University
Portland, Oregon

Preface

I wrote this book because, while my mother's descent into Alzheimer's disease was excruciatingly difficult for both of us, I was lucky.

Early on, I met a young woman at church who is a geriatrician.[1] While she could not be Mom's primary care physician she has been a fabulous source of information, is available to me day or night, is endlessly supportive and became a very dear friend. She and her husband had a baby girl the month before I signed Mom up for hospice. After visiting Mom, I would go to her house to rock my goddaughter, which, I am sure, helped to keep me sane. There is something magically restorative about new life, particularly when juxtaposed with end-stage Alzheimer's disease.

I have another friend, a lawyer who is also a nurse, who works for the Oregon Nursing Home

---

1   A geriatrician is a medical doctor who specializes in treating older people.

Association. She provided very valuable information to me and fabulous advice, also very early on. She, too, is always available.

Mom had the good fortune to be accepted as a patient by the geriatrician in town who is held in such high esteem and is so busy that she was no longer accepting new patients. But she agreed to take Mom. This doctor is marvelous, and she always returns phone calls!

When Mom's behavior became violent, when she sat and sobbed all day, when it became impossible to take her out of the memory care residence because she no longer knew me or knew how to sit in a car, a geriatric psychiatrist began making house calls to the memory care residence where she lived. He made her life so much better that I will be grateful to him forever.

I'm a lawyer, so I am able to deal with legal problems. I'm adept at cutting through red tape, asking questions, and getting answers. I have a lot of experience handling difficult people and unpleasant situations.

I was very lucky.

And yet, although I had far more advantages and resources available to me than most people have, ushering my mother through Alzheimer's disease has been terribly difficult. This journey my mother and I have been on has been a huge challenge and a big education. I have learned a lot. I wish I knew at the beginning of this road what I know now.

Even before Mom was diagnosed with Alzheimer's disease, I read many books about Alzheimer's. But no book told me how *actually* to get my mother to go to the dentist when she refused to go. No book warned me about the awful things my mother would say to me or encouraged me that the kindness of absolute strangers would stagger me. No book assured me that, in the midst of the devastation of Alzheimer's disease, there would still be joyful moments for me and for my mother.

So I have written this book for the adult children of those who have Alzheimer's disease. I've included all the things I've learned, all the strategies I've used, all the tips I have, all the things I wish I'd known fifteen years ago. This book is short because adult children who have a parent with Alzheimer's disease don't have time to read long books. They're too busy trying to get from one moment to the next, from one crisis to the next, one day at a time.

Every time I thought it couldn't get any worse, it did. But I have been astonished at the moments of joy. This is a long and difficult journey, but I will treasure the happy moments Mom and I have had along the way.

I hope this book makes the road easier for others.

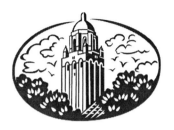

Phyllis

My mother, Phyllis, was born in 1927 in southern California. She attended public elementary school and private high school, where she played volleyball, and went on to Stanford University for three years of undergraduate training before entering Stanford Law School. In 1950, my mother graduated from Stanford Law School, one of three women in her class.

My father, a classmate at Stanford Law School, and Mom were married during their last year of law school and moved north to Portland, Oregon after graduation. Mom passed the Oregon State Bar and worked as a title examiner (the early fifties were not kind to women lawyers) until she had the first of three children in 1952, when she stopped working outside the home.

As her children grew, Phyllis became very involved in volunteer work and was treasurer, then president of the Portland Junior League. Every Thursday night she took modern dance classes and later even taught modern dance at a school for abused and emotionally disturbed girls. A sometime golfer, she was happier playing tennis and enjoyed occasional roles as a member of a children's improvisational theatre group. The witch in Hansel and Gretel was her favorite role, with the grandmother in the same production a close second. She read voraciously all of the time. An excellent bridge player, for nearly forty years she was a member of a bridge club that stopped playing bridge after twenty years because there were so many other interesting things to discuss. Mom tolerated family camping trips (although they weren't her first choice) but loved the family trips to a guest ranch in Canada where she could ride horses. She loved cats and always had at least one, often two.

In the early 1970s, she and my father divorced when their kids were all teenagers. Brushing off her resume was challenging but Mom did so with aplomb and went to work as the founding director of a local nonprofit organization that matched up volunteers with organizations that needed volunteers. Always, Mom loved working because she enjoyed the people she worked with and all the interesting people she met. Four years after her divorce, on her birthday a friend introduced Mom to a friend of his from Rotary. Her friend photocopied his friend's page out of the Rotary telephone directory with his friend's picture on it, folded it into an origami boat and wrote across the hull "This guy will really rock your boat!"

Indeed he did and he and Mom were married one year later to the day on her birthday. Mom and her second husband enjoyed frequent trips to England and Mexico. They were very active members of their church and played tennis together for many years.

At the age of sixty-five, having won dozens of honors during her nearly twenty year career, Mom retired and began volunteering again in earnest. After years of working she was thrilled finally to have time to volunteer as a member of the Citizen Review Board, which advocates for the rights of abused or neglected children and helps delinquent youths become productive members of society. For many years she was recording secretary for a book club that met at a local college as she once again had time to read several books a week. Although her Thursday night dance class ended in the 1970s, after she retired she regularly walked several miles a day most days through her neighborhood.

In the mid-1990s, Mom was diagnosed with esophageal cancer. She was given less than thirteen months to live and was treated with chemotherapy but has now survived for more than eleven years.

My mother was a brilliant woman. In her youth and young adulthood she excelled academically at all levels of her education and continued to read avidly throughout her life. The first comment anyone who knew my mother would make to me, upon discovering that I was her daughter, was "Your mother is such a smart woman!" Volunteering was a defining part of her personality and she was committed to using her time and talents for the benefit of community in which she lived.

As I write this book, Mom has end-stage Alzheimer's disease. At this point, my mother—who was so active most of her life—is unable to move, except to cross her legs, one knee over another, and to occasionally move her hand to scratch her face or tap her toes to music. Her days are spent confined to a wheel chair, a recliner, or bed. Too disabled to feed herself, she can eat only food that has been pureed and strained. Unable to speak an intelligible word she still struggles occasionally to make herself understood. Although I believe she can still sense when family or caregivers are nearby, she is blind. She has one friend from her past who continues to visit her occasionally.

Mom still has excellent hearing, recognizes the voices of her favorite caregivers and responds to them from forty feet away. She enjoys listening to music and sometimes sings along. Never a touchy kind of woman, now she enjoys having her hands rubbed with lotion and sometimes enjoys holding hands. A hardcore coffee-drinker all of her adult life, she always hated anything coffee-flavored like coffee ice cream or lattes but now she likes frappuccinos. A wonderful, young hospice volunteer visits her every week and reads mystery stories to her. Mom loves listening to the cadence of her voice.

To the astonishment of everyone—her doctors and children alike— she lives on, long past every prognosis for either her cancer or Alzheimer's disease.

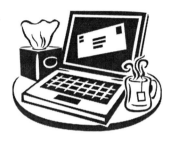

Chapter 1: Early Stage

I remember that ominous feeling I had when I began to wonder if maybe Mom had Alzheimer's disease.[2] We all forget things, we all get confused, we all have bad days when we become angrier than the situation merits. Probably every sibling has called another sibling and voiced concerns about how a parent is doing, even talked about whether the parent is slipping mentally or perhaps has Alzheimer's. Most adult children do not live with their parents; most of us haven't had experience with Alzheimer's disease, so most of us don't recognize the symptoms.[3]

2   Alzheimer's disease is a progressive, degenerative disease that attacks the brain and results in impaired memory, thinking, and behavior. Alzheimer's Association handout, undated.

3   The symptoms of Alzheimer's disease include 1) loss of memory, 2) loss of intellectual ability severe enough to interfere with routine work or social activities,

When you get to the stage that you are talking fairly regularly with siblings about how Mom or Dad is doing, begin keeping notes. Include dates or, at least, list a month and year. You think you will remember when Mom or Dad first started acting oddly, but you won't. You'll find yourself having to backtrack to remember which year a certain behavior started. You're not keeping track of dates to humiliate your parent or to be mean; you're keeping track because this information will be important to the doctors later and you'll need to be able to remind yourself of the incidents if your parent is reluctant to seek treatment. And you're keeping track because you will want to forget about the behavior because no one wants a parent to have Alzheimer's disease.

It used to be that there wasn't anything that could be done about Alzheimer's disease so there was no reason to have conversations early with a parent you suspected had Alzheimer's. Now, we have

---

3) changes in personality, 4) changes in mood and behavior, 5) language problems, such as trouble finding words 6) problems with abstract thinking, 7) poor or decreased judgment, 8) disorientation in place and time. Alzheimer's Association handout, undated. The loss of memory of Alzheimer's disease isn't the forgetfulness of losing your car keys; it's forgetting what your keys are for. It is the memory loss of making the same phone call to the same person for the same reason several times in a short period of time, like ten minutes.

early interventions that are very helpful so there are compelling reasons to talk with your parent and to seek treatment as soon as possible.

It's never easy for children to talk with a parent about forgetfulness, although some parents are more receptive to their children's comments and concerns than others. Be aware that one of the aspects of Alzheimer's which many people don't know about is mood change. People with Alzheimer's can have huge mood swings. The most even-tempered parent may lash out in a ferocious manner. It's wise to be prepared to be attacked verbally during this discussion.

If your parent refuses to discuss your concerns with you or you are unable to convince your parent to see a doctor, consider having a family meeting and inviting a trusted family friend. While the discussion may be successful, consider carefully that it may be unsuccessful, as well. Consider whether one sibling should bear the brunt of the anger, leaving the rest of the siblings to help get things done on other occasions. The approach that worked for our family was to have one sibling—me, because I lived in the same city as our mother—be the one who took the heat. When I was totally unsuccessful, I would call in my sister and brother. While Mom spent a year furiously angry with me, as a family we were able to accomplish a lot with this "good cop, bad cop" approach. To our very great advantage, my brother could accomplish things with Mom that neither my sister nor I could: he was able to talk her into moving into the retirement center; we were able to convince Mom to give him her power of attorney so he could handle her finances; and, after many discussions, he took away her car keys. I called him my walk-on-water brother because he could be successful when I failed.

The most important goal of these discussions is to get your parent to a doctor who can diagnose and treat the dementia.[4] Second, at some point it will be helpful for your parent to talk with a lawyer to make certain that end-of-life planning is complete, to prepare a will or estate plan, to give power of attorney to a trusted sibling or friend, and—very importantly—to complete a health-care power of attorney. Third, in the best of all worlds, your parent could be involved in making decisions about where to live during late-stage Alzheimer's, when living independently is no longer an option, and how best to pay for care.

To address the issues Alzheimer's disease raises early on in the disease is hugely beneficial. There are great benefits in finding a good doctor for your parent early in the disease and in being organized and prepared. But, many families have to wait for a crisis because the parent is unwilling or, because of the damage to the brain that the disease has already caused, is unable to talk about these issues.

---

4   Alzheimer's disease is only one of over sixty types of dementia illnesses, which can produce similar symptoms. Different types of dementias are treated differently. Some can be treated effectively.

Those whose parents refuse to discuss their forgetfulness will find it nerve wracking to wait for the crisis, but there are things you can do to help prepare.

Tips

1. When you first begin to notice odd behavior, start keeping notes. Include at least the month and year and a description of the behavior.
2. Communicate with your family. I found that e-mail made this easy because I didn't have to have the same conversation twice. By e-mailing both my brother and sister at the same time, the three of us could communicate easily and effectively most of the time. Try to come to a consensus about the best strategy to approach your parent.
3. Talk with your parent. Get to know your mother or father's health-care providers, religious advisers and friends. Encourage your parent to give health-care providers permission to talk with you about health issues affecting your parent.

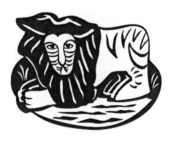

Chapter 2: Waiting for the Crisis

Lucky families are able to talk with the parent who is showing signs of dementia and make plans for the time when the dementia becomes so bad that some sort of intervention is necessary. Oftentimes, and some folks who are knowledgeable about Alzheimer's disease and other dementias say *most* often, families have to wait for a crisis. A crisis is more than a pattern of disturbing events or a single event of even moderate magnitude, such as your parent becoming disoriented returning home from the grocery store but ultimately arriving safely. A crisis is a cataclysmic event that suddenly changes everything.

We knew that we were approaching that crisis. Mom refused to talk about her forgetfulness and would become furious if we mentioned it, which seemed odd to us. She had erratic behavior. One

Christmas, she called to see if I would bring the quiches to Christmas brunch. I said yes and we chatted for a few minutes. One minute after we hung up, she called again, and we had the same conversation. And a minute after we hung up from that conversation, she called again, and we had the conversation again. Once, when she and her husband came to dinner, she brought me a small, carved lion which she had found in her basement and she thought was mine. I told her it wasn't, but she became angry and insisted that she knew it was.[5] When I asked her to put the dinner salads on the table, she became very upset that she couldn't remember where they belonged on the table.

We tried, again and again, to talk with our stepfather about Mom's dementia; but he wouldn't meet with us or talk with us about it. He said he felt that he would be betraying his wife to talk about her behind her back. Although he gave us occasional bulletins about her forgetfulness and her crying, he couldn't bring himself to get serious about these discussions. He said that she would lose her car in the parking lot at the grocery store, or get lost on the way home, and would backtrack to the store and call him. Among ourselves, my siblings and I discussed that we would be in big trouble if anything happened to him.

---

5   For several years, I kept the lion in the garden window by my kitchen sink to remind me to be patient.

I did do a few things. I went to the Alzheimer's Association Web site and tried to learn more about Alzheimer's disease. I tried to convince Mom to take me along to her appointments with her doctors. At one point, she agreed to be tested for Alzheimer's disease and told us that the doctor said she was "predementia" but never mentioned the word Alzheimer's. She vehemently objected to my talking with her doctor.

I met with her husband's adult children, and we tried a different approach. They were able to convince their dad to look at retirement living situations and get him and Mom on a waiting list at a local independent living apartment complex, but the waiting list for the kind of apartment they wanted was years long.

Then Mom's husband had a stroke, for which he needed a lengthy hospitalization and rehabilitation. Mom couldn't live alone but refused to have anyone live with her. So the crisis was upon us.

Looking back, there were a few more things I could have done while we waited for the crisis. I wish I had written a letter to Mom's doctors and dentist[6] telling them how concerned we all were about her and why. Once we were in crisis, her medical professionals met with me and shared her medical information. Their rationale was that Mom's husband was now disabled, and they were all grateful to have a family

---

6   Mom had a long history of dental issues but liked her dentist very much. His office staff worked hard to enable me to continue taking Mom in for dental work for as along as I could.

member to speak with. I was chagrined at the number of times I heard how long they'd been worried about Mom; yet none of them had picked up the phone to call me, even though I was listed in their medical information as a person to call in the event of an emergency. Perhaps a letter would have jostled one of them to the phone. Even though Mom would have been furious with me, I might have been willing to pay that price, had I known then what I know now about how helpful early intervention can be.

While HIPPA[7] now prohibits medical professionals from giving any information about a patient to nearly anyone without the patient's consent, there's no prohibition about giving information *to* the medical professional. So, while I was dealing with Mom's doctors in a pre-HIPPA era, I think the same general approach would work today.

I also wish I had initiated contact with her minister and her close friends. After the crisis, when I did call these folks, I heard that they, too, had long been very worried about Mom but had been reluctant to call me. The risk, of course, is that Mom would

---

7   HIPPA is the Health Insurance Portability and Accountability Act of 1996 (which became effective after April 2003). It is federal legislation that, among other things, regulates to whom medication information can be given about a patient. As a general matter, no information about any adult can be given to anyone unless that adult has consented in writing.

have been furious with me for contacting them—and perhaps with them for talking to me, too. While that would have been unpleasant, it might have been a catalyst for sooner action. She spent over a year being furious with me, anyway. If we'd been able to get her help sooner, it might have been worth her additional anger.

Tips

1. Go to the Alzheimer's Association Web site,[8] and to your local Alzheimer's Association office, to learn all you can about Alzheimer's and other dementias.

2. Consider sending a letter to your parent's doctors describing your concerns. Consider also contacting your parent's religious adviser and good friends to tell them how concerned you are.

3. Keep talking to your parent about health issues. Try to address as many of the important issues— getting a health-care power of attorney in place, planning where to live, sorting through financial and legal matters—resolved as you can before the crisis, because surely the crisis will come.

---

8   www.alz.org. There are many Web sites that provide information about Alzheimer's disease, which you can find through any Internet search engine.

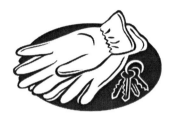

Chapter 3: Middle Stage

Mom was beyond merely confused. We all knew that something horrible was going on, but she couldn't talk about her memory loss without getting terribly angry. Looking back, I know now that her anger was both face saving and the progress of the mood-altering part of Alzheimer's. My siblings and I knew when Mom's husband had a stroke that we were in crisis.

Mom couldn't stay alone. We were concerned that she wasn't locking doors and that she left burners on. We knew that, when she drove to the store, the one she'd driven to for fifty years, she sometimes lost the car in the parking lot or got lost on the way home. We knew she couldn't remember how to cook anymore and that she was unable to find her way to the hospital to visit her husband.

She wouldn't let me stay overnight with her. For the first several nights, one of my stepsisters stayed with her, and we quickly moved Mom into a retirement center. But we couldn't move her directly into assisted living because the retirement complex Mom and her husband had chosen required that each new resident initially move into independent living.[9] So, we had to move Mom into independent living.

While we felt marginally more secure with Mom living in an apartment in a retirement complex, we still had huge issues to face because Mom was so disabled. She had to learn to go down to the dining room for meals. We put up signs in her apartment that listed the times of meals, and I got her a wrist bracelet key chain that she could wear so she wouldn't lose the key to her room. My sister printed the directions to the dining room on one side of an index card and the directions back from the dining room to her apartment on the other side, laminated it, and attached it to the key chain. That way, Mom always had directions to her apartment and the dining room with her. At mealtimes, I would call to remind her to go downstairs to eat.

I got her a telephone with speed dial and entered our names and phone numbers so that she could push the button by the name to contact us, without

---

9   In independent living, residents live on their own, perhaps taking meals in a dining room. In assisted living, there is on-call twenty-four-hour help to assist residents in emergencies, and often there are additional services available (for an extra fee) such as a med-aide to give medication or caregivers to assist with bathing and other needs.

having to remember our phone numbers. The phone was only marginally successful. I don't think she ever understood that pushing only one button dialed a whole phone number.

Each apartment had a small stove with a lid that could be closed to make a countertop. Mom would boil water for tea or coffee and leave the burner on. After much thought, I took the knobs to the burners off the stove and told her they were lost. While I commiserated with her about how long it was taking the maintenance man to come to replace the knobs, in actuality I had hidden them up high on the top of the cabinet.[10] After about a week, I closed the lid, and she forgot that the stove was there.

While I worried a little that she would go for a walk and get lost, generally Mom was fearful, and I thought she was unlikely to venture out on her own. Still, if she *were* to leave the retirement center, she would have no idea how to get back, and historically she had loved strolling around her neighborhood. So, I signed Mom up on the Safe Return program. This

---

10 This was the first time I actually lied to Mom. While I always tried to be honest, I eventually reluctantly concluded that it was impossible always to tell the entire truth to Mom. Often the unvarnished truth confused or frightened her or made her miserable. I finally decided that my priorities were to keep her safe and as happy as I could and that I would be less than truthful, when I needed to and thought I could get away with it, to achieve my priorities.

is a fabulous program offered by a subsidiary of the Alzheimer's Association. For a small fee, I registered Mom by sending in her name, a description, a picture, her address, and my name and address. They sent back two bracelets (or you can get dog tags) with the Alzheimer's Association logo on the front and the notation "Memory Impaired" on the back and "To help Phyllis call 1-800-572-1122," together with an identifying number. Law enforcement people know to look for the bracelet or dog tag when they find a person who doesn't know where they live. In fact, anyone could call the 800 number. While I was never able to convince Mom to wear the bracelet, I hid one in her purse and took comfort that some law enforcement agencies know to call the 800 number even if they don't find a bracelet or tag. Safe Return might be able to identify Mom by area of town and description. I figured that if Mom were missing, I would know and could call Safe Return to see if anyone had been found, even if Mom didn't have the bracelet on.

I once asked Mom if she ever went walking. She said she wanted to, but that the woman at the front desk of the building told her that it was against the rules for her to go out alone. While I knew this wasn't the rule, since this makeshift system seemed to be working, I left it alone.

These were hard settling-in days. I told Mom that it was too far for her to drive to see her husband so I took her every day. Mom decided that she couldn't go anywhere without her blue fleece gloves. Even on sunny days, even in the middle of summer, she would only leave with her blue fleece gloves. And, of course, she was always losing them. When we went to coffee or a store, she would leave one some haphazard place, and we would spend what seemed like hours looking for them. Or she would leave the apartment without them, and we would have to go back for them. I came to hate the blue fleece gloves. At every turn, they annoyed me. It took me several months before I had the epiphany that I had to be responsible for the gloves. Instead of resenting and hating them, I had to manage them: I had to know where they were at all times. If I remembered to look for them every minute or so, then I wouldn't need to spend hours looking for them when she lost them. So, I put them on my radar: I learned to check every minute or two for the blue fleece gloves. And then, because Mom always had them with her, perhaps because she never felt like she lost them, they slowly ceased to be an issue.

Once Mom was moved and safe, we embarked on a series of visits to doctors to have her dementia diagnosed. On September 12, 2001, I picked her up to take her to the appointment to see a specialist in dementia. As she got into the car, she said, "We don't have to be sorry about all those people who were killed because it happened a very, very long time ago," referring to the terrorist attacks on the World Trade Center the day before. I knew we were in deep trouble.

We spent much of the day at a clinic where both she and I were interviewed and she was given a complete physical. The physician in charge told me that he was amazed that she had been able to cope so well for so long, that she must have been a very smart woman.[11] By the end of the month, she had been diagnosed with middle-stage Alzheimer's disease.[12]

During middle-stage Alzheimer's, the most difficult times were when I had to convince my

---

11 Mom not only was a very smart woman, but she was very strong willed and fought Alzheimer's disease every step of the way. People who are quite intelligent often are diagnosed later in the disease because they've developed strategies to compensate for many of the symptoms of Alzheimer's.

12 Middle-stage Alzheimer's is characterized by increasing memory loss and confusion and a shorter attention span. Look for problems recognizing close friends or family; repetitive statements and/or movements; occasional muscle twitches or jerking; problems finding the right words or organizing thoughts; loss of impulse control, fear of bathing, and trouble dressing. Families need to consider these issues as well as anticipate the problems of wandering, getting lost, and an increasing inability to care for self—like bathing or teeth brushing. Administration of medication becomes a major issue because there are good medications available to help slow the progress of Alzheimer's—but only if the patient *takes* the medication. By middle stage, patients cannot administer their own medication.

mother to go along with something that she didn't want to do. For instance, at first I had a lot of trouble convincing Mom to let me go into the examining room at the doctor or dental office with her. We were at an impasse. Because of her Alzheimer's, no medical professional would see her without me in the examining room, but she didn't want to let me accompany her to the see the doctor. So, when the medical assistant called her name for her appointment, I would get up to accompany her, and she would order me to stay in the waiting room. Ultimately what worked best was a combination of statement and distraction: "Mom, you know we've discussed me meeting this doctor, so I'll come in just long enough to shake his hand. Oh, my goodness, look at this fabulous bouquet of spring flowers on this desk! It is just lovely and has your very favorite daffodils in it! Come, look!" I found if I talked fast, I could get out of the waiting room and down the hall into the examining room with her. So long as I kept talking and walking, she would follow. At one appointment, she said, "I know you're distracting me to get into that room," which broke my heart.

The primary difficulty with this approach is that it made me look like an overbearing daughter, or worse. But, what mattered was that I made it to the examining room so Mom could have her appointment with the doctor. Once the doctor arrived and greeted both of us, Mom was much happier to have me there to talk with the doctor. I don't think she wanted to talk to the doctor alone, but neither did she want me with her.

Oddly enough, the unrelenting progress of Alzheimer's solved this problem. As Mom's Alzheimer's progressed, it became more and more obvious to everyone in the waiting room that she had dementia. On more than one occasion, when I was near tears, trying to handle Mom, someone would lean over and tell me that their grandmother had Alzheimer's and that they understood the problem and my anguish.

So, amazingly enough, for awhile it became easier to take her many places because, although she was often difficult, people knew just by looking at her that she had Alzheimer's and, almost without exception, were very kind. If Mom barged to the front of a line, others in the line gave way to her and smiled at me. If I was trying to wait in line to pay for coffee and Mom started to wander away, people offered to let me go before them, and in one instance offered to pay for the coffee. Strangers would smile at me in a knowing manner. I was astonished at the kindness of strangers.

Soon after Mom got used to having me in the examining room to talk with her doctor, another problem developed. She refused to go to the doctor or dentist at all.

At first I fell back on the old standby of distraction. I could distract her by arranging something happy before the appointment. I began to understand the guiding rule of dementia: If Mom was happy and laughing, I could accomplish almost anything. If she was unhappy, I was sunk. We would go out for coffee and to watch the ice skaters at the local mall, which she loved. Then we would walk through the local discount shop and look at clothes and swing by the unpleasant appointment on the way back to her apartment.

If distraction didn't work, sometimes agreeing with her would give me the foothold I needed to convince her to go. A friend of mine, who works in the geriatric health care field, told me as soon as Mom was diagnosed with Alzheimer's that I would never win another argument with her. "Think about it, Anne," she said. "You cannot possibly ever win by arguing. Don't even try." It was very wise advice. So, if Mom didn't want to go to the doctor, I'd say, "Well, he's your doctor. I think he's a jerk. I wouldn't want to see him either, but he said you had to come back in today. I'd be perfectly happy not seeing him today, so how about if we fire him and I find someone better?"[13] Then, of course, she would defend her doctor and see him more happily.

However, there were some days when there was lots of fuss. I found that, for my own sanity, I had to break each appointment down into little bits and

---

13 This approach worked with the internist she was seeing when I became responsible for her heath care. After we switched to her geriatrician, I wouldn't use it because Mom's geriatrician was a fabulous woman whom Mom and I both liked very much.

tackle each bit one at a time. If I worried about the entire event at once, I would get so stressed that Mom would sense it, and we would lose her all-important good mood. So, my first goal would be to get her in the car, which I could do with the promise of a trip to the mall. After visiting the mall, she would be ready to go home, so she would get in the car without a fuss.

The next bit would be to drive her to the appointment. I played soothing classical music in the car and kept up a running commentary of hilarious stories about my children or my sister's children or my childhood. I didn't need an endless supply of such stories, because Mom would forget them. I had about a dozen stories that I would tell, recalling each one as if she had never heard it before and laughing hysterically, which would make her laugh, too. I'd comment about the people and lovely gardens that we drove by. Sometimes she would tumble to the fact that we were going someplace she didn't want to go and threaten to get out of the car. Then I would keep my finger on the electronic "lock" button in the car to keep her from opening the door in traffic, chattering all the while, searching for some topic that would break her train of thought. I became adept at free association and asking her questions about her childhood or her old college roommates.

The most challenging part of taking her to appointments would be getting her out of the car and into the appointment. There was not much I could have done if she just flat refused to leave the car, but it never actually came to that. Sometimes, taking a friend along was helpful, because Mom still felt the social pressure to behave well around a stranger.

Once, on the way to the dentist for a tooth extraction, I worried that my luck was finally up. While she liked her dentist, she hated dental work and had said she wouldn't go into his office. I hoped the entire way there for a diversion to get Mom out of the car, and I was worried enough that I had taken a friend along to help. As we arrived in the parking lot, along a busy street in a business area that bordered a residential neighborhood, Mom said again that she wouldn't get out of the car. As I pulled into the parking lot, a big, beautiful tabby cat walked leisurely across the lot. "Oh, look, a kitty!" I said. "I wonder if she'll let us pet her?" Mom popped out of the car before I even had it parked. After petting the cat, I led the way, and my friend walked so closely behind Mom that Mom had no choice but to follow or my friend would bump into her. Once again, distraction was the key. By breaking Mom's train of thought, by turning her thoughts to something that she loved and made her happy, I was able to accomplish what needed to be done. When the dental assistant called her name, all three of us (Mom, my friend and I) stood up, but Mom turned to exit to the parking lot. I took her hand, and my friend followed immediately behind her as we led her to the dental chair just as we had led her through the parking lot. My friend and I each knelt by the dental chair, stroking Mom's hands as I told stories about my childhood to keep her laughing.

Another time, Mom needed new lingerie. I found a lingerie shop where I could make an appointment ahead of time to take Mom in for a fitting. I went to the shop, met the owners, and explained the situation about Mom. I talked to Mom about the trip and presented it as an exciting adventure, but Mom wasn't buying it. On the way to the appointment, she figured out where we were going and threatened to get out of the car, but I kept my finger on the lock button and kept on talking. As we pulled up to the store, she retreated to one of her safe harbors: "I've been here before," she said. Although I knew she had never been to the store, I was quick to respond, "Then I'm sure you loved these ladies as much as I do. I'm sure your favorite saleslady will be there today!" She jumped out of the car eagerly, because she thought she was on familiar territory.

During middle-stage Alzheimer's, Mom frequently said that she had done before something that we knew she had never done at all. She was convinced that she had lived before in the retirement center where she moved. At first, I told her that she was mistaken: it seemed cruel to agree with her when I knew it wasn't true. She became furious. Once I danced around it. I said that the center was so lovely that it must remind her of a hotel where she had stayed once. That irritated her because it implied that she was confused.

Eventually, I discovered the wisdom of my friend's warning that I would never win an argument with a person with Alzheimer's, and I learned to say, "Then aren't we lucky that you were able to get your old apartment back!"

Sometimes, however, absolute honesty was the way to go. I remember the day that I had to tell Mom that we were moving her from independent living to assisted living, because she was too disabled to live without twenty-four-hour supervision. The apartment in assisted living was smaller than the one in independent living and looked out onto an asphalt rooftop, instead of the beautiful downtown skyline and river view she had in her other apartment. I knew she would hate everything about the new apartment and that she would hate being told that she needed more help or accepting any help at all. There was nothing good about the situation, and I was expecting another huge scene. Since there was no way to sugarcoat the news or avoid her reaction to it, I just gave it to her straight. Together, we met with the head of the assisted living section and made all the arrangements for her to move in, even before she saw the apartment. Then I told her that she was going to hate the apartment because it was small and had no view but that simply was the way that things had to be right now. I told her that she might eventually like living on the assisted living floor because there were more people to talk to, but they might bug her too much and she might hate that too. If she didn't learn to like it, we would move her again as soon as we could; but, in the meantime, she would hate it. Then, as the meeting ended, I said, "So, now would you like to see this apartment that you're going to love to hate?" And she started to laugh. Occasionally, being brutally honest worked best.

Eventually, I learned that a good mood was my most important ally, even if it easily could be lost. By the end of middle-stage Alzheimer's, Mom was living in memory care and some days would sit and sob piteously. We tried hard to help her mood with medication, but the medication process takes time. One day she and I were walking down the hallway after having had a wonderful time in the garden. Mom was laughing and happy. As we approached one resident's room, we could hear the resident, Flora, crying. Mom stopped laughing. As we got closer, Mom began to cry. As we passed by the room and turned the corner, where we couldn't hear Flora crying anymore, Mom stopped crying, too. Anxious to restore the mood, I reminded Mom what a great time we'd just had, how beautiful the flowers were, and that we could go back out tomorrow. By the time we reached the end of the hallway, she was happy again. Flora's crying had destroyed Mom's good mood, but by then I knew how to restore it. I'd learned that mood was king and what I needed to do to serve the king.

Middle-stage Alzheimer's was a very difficult stage; perhaps it is the most difficult stage. I'm not sure that I realized at the time, though, that it was just one stage of Alzheimer's. Sometimes I felt we would be in it forever. But the disease marches slowly onward. I found Mom's blue fleece gloves, the ones that had plagued me so, in her drawer, stuffed all the way to the back and forgotten, nearly a year after she had been confined to a wheelchair, unable to walk or feed herself. They had lost their power. And when I looked at my mom, in a nearly vegetative state with late-stage Alzheimer's, I almost missed those days of looking for the blue fleece gloves.

Tips

1. Never, ever argue with a person with Alzheimer's disease. You will never win the argument—even if you do, they will forget—and you will lose the good mood you need. Find some other way to accomplish your objective. Although I never tried to physically force Mom to do something she didn't want to do, I know that approach would have been unsuccessful and dangerous for both her and for me.

2. There will come a point when you no longer can remind your parent to do things, or help them to do things yourself. Recognize that point and do whatever needs to be done for them, even without their knowing you've undertaken to help them. I found if I quietly took responsibility for the gloves, they were no longer an issue.

3.   Break down large tasks into manageable smaller bits—for your parent with dementia but also for yourself. People with dementia respond to mood—particularly your mood—and if you're totally stressed out, your parent will sense it, and that will destroy his or her mood.

4.   Use humor or distraction to keep the mood happy. Once you lose the good mood, you won't accomplish anything until you get the good mood back.

5.   Try to be honest.

6.   Consider whether you will be willing to equivocate or tell less then the truth to your parent before you find yourself in the moment when you may find that telling the absolute truth to be so detrimental to what needs to be done that you don't want to tell it. I thought a long time before I began fudging the truth to Mom, and Mom was very disabled before I thought I could get away with half-truths. Ultimately, though, I decided it was necessary for her happiness and well-being. When the day came that I told my first half-truth to her, I was at peace with my decision so I was able to get away with it and, as a result, preserve her good mood.

7.   Use every diversion to your benefit; learn to create diversions when you need them.

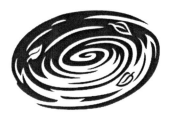

Chapter 4: How Bad Can It Get?

How bad can the situation really get with a parent with Alzheimer's? For months and months on end, I thought I had hit bottom with Mom, that it couldn't get any worse. And it always did.

The bad times began slowly, as angry outbursts at me when I tried to talk with her about her memory loss, and then accelerated into more public displays. During one visit to the local mall with Mom, I made the mistake of taking my two sons, then ages eleven and twelve, trying to combine an outing Mom loved with an opportunity for the boys to get new athletic shoes. Mom became so angry at me (I cannot remember now what she was angry about) that she had me near tears. My twelve-year-old son physically placed himself between me and Mom, put his arm around me, and said, "Mom, that's the Alzheimer's talking, not Grandma Phyl." I never took the boys out in public with her again.

I learned that day that it never worked to take Mom anywhere and have any agenda other than her. It was impossible to do anything else when I was with her because she was so unpredictable and erratic that she required constant supervision. When I was with Mom, she required all my attention.

I wish I had known when I began to care for Mom that she would turn on me one day and scream, "I hope you get Alzheimer's disease and die." If someone had told me, I would have dismissed the warning, sure that this would never happen, because Mom had never said hurtful or hateful things to any of us. But I would have been alerted, and I think that caution would have guarded my heart just a little so that the day that she shrieked those words would have been a little easier. Instead, her words blindsided me and scored a direct hit. I went home and vomited three times. She, of course, forgot.

Mom was angry at me that day because I had taken away her ability to regulate her own medicines by hiring the nursing staff at the retirement center where she lived to give them to her each day. She was unable to remember to take them herself; and her only hope to remain in independent living, rather than move to assisted living, was to take her medications regularly. She desperately wanted to remain in independent living, and I was hoping to help her stay there for a few more months. But from her standpoint, I had taken away what was left of her independence, and she fought back the only way she could, as damaged as her brain was by Alzheimer's disease. I knew all that on that day, but I was unprepared for her naked fury and hate. I thought she was going to hit me (another thing that she had never done). On top of being devastated, I was horrified that she would wish the disease that was going to kill her on her daughter. Looking back, I wonder if I might not have been so devastated if I hadn't been so shocked. Perhaps I wouldn't have been so shocked if I had been warned.

We moved her into a memory care residence eighteen months later, and she stuck out her tongue at me and screamed, "I hate you, I hate you and I hope you die!" By then, I had learned to listen to what she was feeling instead of to her words—and to let the words bounce off me. I had learned a lot more about Alzheimer's and how to manage Mom. That day, I knew she was really saying that she hated her situation, hated being moved, hated that things were changing, and hated being afraid. I responded, "I know you're mad at me, and I don't blame you. Let's sit down and have a glass of wine and some cheese and crackers, and you can tell me all the other reasons you hate me because I know there must be more." After she had several glasses of wine (that was actually grape juice), and I had only had one (because I'm driving, I told her), I was able to help her calm down. I was able to distract her with the "wine" and cheese.

We talked about why she was angry. I assured her that she was safe and I would stay with her for a long time. I talked and talked and talked. She gradually forgot her fury. Slowly, I was able to change the mood.

The sad truth is that now, with Mom in end-stage Alzheimer's, I cheer at any coherent thought. For instance, when she was in late stage, Mom hated to be walked. It took two people to assist her to walk even a very short distance, and she often screamed or cried out that she was being burned. One day after the caregivers had walked her to a recliner, then left to assist other residents, I was tucking her lap blanket around her as she continued to fuss for several minutes. She looked right at me and said very sternly, "You are a big dope—the king of dopes!" and I was absolutely thrilled. An entire, appropriate sentence, which expressed exactly what she thought, was a huge gift to me. I called the caregivers back, and we marveled, quietly, away from Mom so she couldn't hear us, at the determination, willpower, and thought it took to get that one sentence out through the tangled proteins of Alzheimer's that have clogged her mind.

As the disease progresses and plateaus, then progresses again, there will be high points and low points. There will bad times when you least expect them. The night that I got a call from the memory care residence that reported that Mom had hit another resident, knocked a woman who was four inches taller and thirty-five pounds heavier than herself to the floor, was a bad night for me. At some level, I might expect a call from the school principal that one of my sons was in a fight; but to get a call that my mother had knocked Victoria to the floor—and to feel that I was expected to have some sort of solution or response—was mind-boggling to me. It was such a reversal of the circle of life that it took me greatly by surprise.

I felt, somehow, like it was my fault that Mom hit Victoria. I know this is irrational, but I've seen the same reaction in other family members. We feel like our parents, who have advanced dementia, should be behaving properly and that it's our responsibility if they don't. On top of feeling guilty, I was embarrassed and horrified, and I didn't have the faintest idea what to do. And even worse, I knew that I had to solve this problem or Mom might have to move.

But there are new strategies at each low point. The day that Mom knocked Victoria to the floor was one of the times that it was invaluable to have a geriatrician on my team. Drugs were the only effective tool against her violent behavior, and eventually we needed help from a geriatric psychiatrist to balance her medications.

It's very important to pass on these bad times, as odd as that sounds. One day as I was arriving to visit Mom, the daughter of another resident was leaving in tears. I looked inquiringly at a caregiver who took pity on the daughter and said (although perhaps she shouldn't have because of HIPPA), "Her mom hit another resident yesterday." I ran after the woman, caught up with her in the parking lot, and told her about the time that Mom hit Victoria and knocked her to the floor. She needed to know because I knew she was feeling totally and utterly alone. She was caught in that vortex created by the circle of life reversing on itself—the same vortex that sucked me under on the night when I received the phone call that Mom hit Victoria—and she had no idea how to react or what she could possibly do.

I had walked that road, so I understood the depth of her misery. She needed to know that I'd been in that position. She needed to know it wasn't her fault that her mom had hit another resident, and no one thought the less of her—or her mother.[14] Unhappy as she was, she needed to know that I'd cried myself to sleep the night I got the phone call about Mom knocking Victoria to the floor; but the next day, together with Mom's doctors, we'd embarked upon a course of action that proved to be a solution. She needed to know that my mom hadn't hit anyone in months, and she needed the name and phone number

---

14 One of the wonderful things about memory care is that no offense is taken or judgment made because of behavior that would cause offense outside of memory care. The caregivers understand that the residents are unable to control their behavior. Family members of residents learn to take no offense (if only so no one will take offense at the behavior of their resident). And the residents quickly forget any offending behavior.

of the geriatric psychiatrist who'd treated Mom. As I wrote down his name and phone number, I knew that, beyond giving her the name of the man who likely could solve the medical problem her mom faced, I was giving her hope and at least one better night's sleep.

Misery loves company. Sometimes passing along the miserable experience—and the solution you found—is the kindest thing you can do for someone. Every bad experience is a lesson, and after awhile I began to understand that I would survive, that I could learn from even the worst experience and pass the lessons along.

Tips

1. Know that times will get very bad. Know that your parent may say horrible things, but it's the Alzheimer's talking. Guard your heart. Be alert and prepared to hear terrible things.

2. Instead of listening to what your parent says, try to look beyond the words to the emotion that your parent is feeling. Remember that the ability to communicate is seriously compromised in dementia. Even though your parent may still be able to form words and sentences, the area of the brain that controls speech is damaged. Focus on the emotions that your parent's words express, not the words themselves. When you respond, address the emotion—the frustration,

the anger, the fear—not the precise words your parent used.

3. In the same manner that adults should never respond in kind to insulting verbal slings and arrows from children—simply because adults are adults and children are children—remember that your parent has dementia, *but you do not.* Your parent cannot control what your parent says, but you can control what you say in response.[15] Never respond in a hurtful manner to a hurtful statement.

4. Share the bad times. Be alert for the times when others will need to know the bad times you've endured, so that they know that they can endure their own.

5. Consider joining an Alzheimer's support group.[16] It can be a good place not only to share tips but also to share misery. Some days, just to know

---

15 When her mother had early-stage Alzheimer's, a friend of mine made and laminated a card that she kept by her phone that said, in big block letters, "She cannot control what she is saying, but YOU CAN!" She took the card out and set it in front of her every time her mother called.

16 You can find an Alzheimer's support group through your local Alzheimer's Association or check with local memory care facilities. Often there are support groups associated with residences that care for the memory disabled.

that someone else has encountered the problem will help you feel better.

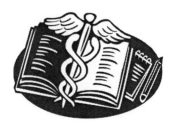

Chapter 5: Dealing with Doctors

The best way to establish a relationship with your parent's doctor is to have your parent cheerfully take you to an appointment with the doctor and give the doctor permission to discuss everything about him or herself with you, any time of the day or night. This is what my husband's parents did, and it worked great.

My mother refused to ever take any of us to her doctors' appointments. Five years before she was diagnosed with Alzheimer's, when she was diagnosed with esophageal cancer, she refused to let me or my siblings even meet her doctor. When I sent a letter to her oncologist expressing our concern, Mom specifically instructed her oncologist to tell us nothing. As a result, when Mom's husband had a stroke, when the crisis hit, none of us had ever met any of Mom's doctors.

I decided that, while she had told her oncologist to tell us nothing, I was aware of nothing that prevented me from giving her doctors information about her. At best, this would give the doctors information I thought they needed, and it would make me feel better that I was doing something, anything, to help. At worst, it would make Mom mad, if she ever found out. But she was already mad at me, and I thought it unlikely that she would ever find out, anyway.

I drafted a letter, addressed to all her doctors, explaining her current circumstances. In the letter, I included all her doctors' names, addresses, and phone numbers (so that they could contact each other easily) as well as the addresses, phone numbers, e-mail addresses, and cell phone numbers of my siblings. At my request, my siblings reviewed and edited my words so I could say that I spoke for all of Mom's children; then I invited the doctors to contact either of my siblings to talk with them if they had any questions they didn't want to direct to me. I faxed the letter to all her doctors and sent it by regular mail, as well.

Next, I sat down with my friend who is a lawyer and also a nurse and works in the field of health care for the elderly. I figured that medical professionals are most comfortable talking with medical professionals and that I needed to learn the right language and buzz words to set Mom's doctors at ease, to encourage them to talk to me. In the case of Mom's internist, who had done a particularly unsatisfactory job of treating Mom, I needed to learn the right buzz words to convince him to refer her to a special geriatric clinic, without any further time spent on my part, or his, so that her dementia could be diagnosed and treatment could begin.

Then I made an appointment with each of her doctors and went without her. I took an additional copy of the letter to all the doctors with me and gave it to the receptionist at the time I checked in, with a note to the doctor that the purpose of the visit was for me to meet the doctor and give the doctor additional information about Mom. Without exception, Mom's doctors met with me, and the meetings went well, even with her internist.[17]

The same process of faxing a letter to the doctor, and taking an additional copy to the appointment to give to the receptionist before seeing the doctor, worked well when I began actually taking Mom to see her doctors. The morning of each doctor's appointment, I faxed an update letter to the doctor and made an extra copy, which I placed in a sealed envelope with the doctor's name and address typed on it so that it looked like an ordinary business letter. (If it looked like a note, Mom would have been suspicious.) As we entered the doctor's office, I would find Mom a seat

---

17 He admitted to me that he had no particular interest in treating geriatric patients, making it easier for me to convince him to transfer her file to a geriatrician.

in the waiting room, and then, as I checked Mom in with the receptionist, I would hand the letter to the receptionist and ask him or her to please give it to the doctor before the appointment. That way I was able to get current information about Mom to the doctor without having to talk about Mom in front of her, which would have been humiliating to Mom.

Once Mom had been diagnosed by a geriatrician as having middle-stage Alzheimer's, I needed to find a doctor to be her physician.[18] Many family practice doctors and internists aren't interested in treating geriatric patients. I started with the list of doctors from the Alzheimer's Association[19] and interviewed them, one by one, until I found one that seemed to be a good fit for Mom. I made these interview appointments in Mom's name and then met with each doctor without Mom to discuss Mom. I paid each doctor his or her standard fee for the time for the interview. While the doctors were surprised to be interviewed, they were honest about whether they were interested in geriatric patients (and I was surprised that many who were on the Alzheimer's

---

18 Mom was diagnosed by a geriatrician in a special clinic set up for diagnosing dementia in the elderly. He didn't see patients on an ongoing basis.

19 The list was available upon request at the local Alzheimer's Association. If you live too far away from the Alzheimer's Association office in your state, the list can be mailed to you.

list had no particular interest in geriatric patients)[20] and were courteous to me. Several offered to care for Mom until I found a geriatrician who was interested in treating her.

The more I learned about Alzheimer's, and the more I talked with internists and family practice physicians, the more convinced I became that I needed a geriatrician for Mom. A geriatrician is a medical doctor who specializes in treating the elderly. When I took care of my grandmother I learned that the symptoms for ordinary illnesses are very different in geriatric patients[21]and that the dosages for drugs can also vary. Huge advances were being made in the treatment of Alzheimer's, but I knew more about them than some of the family practice specialists and internists I was interviewing to find a doctor for Mom. Mom needed not only a specialist but also a

---

20 Before I made the appointment, I always asked the appointment secretary whether the doctor enjoyed treating the elderly. Often, the appointment secretary had no idea, or would simply say that the doctor had many geriatric patients. I do not know why doctors with no interest in treating the elderly were on the Alzheimer's Association's list of doctors.

21 I cared for my grandmother for the ten years before she died and learned, then, that symptoms in the geriatric population are very different. For instance, my grandmother would become psychotic and hallucinate when she had a urinary tract infection, which is a very common reaction among geriatric patients.

doctor who had a calm demeanor and who would be respectful of her even though she was now seriously disabled. For my part, I wanted to find a doctor who not only would treat Mom with compassion but also would return my phone calls, answer my questions and who had an office close enough to where Mom lived that the drive to appointments would be short enough that she wouldn't become agitated. In short, I wanted the perfect doctor.

Eventually, I found a fabulous geriatrician for Mom.[22] I believe that, if you can find one, the best circumstance is to have a geriatrician treating people with Alzheimer's. But, geriatricians can be few and far between—and it can be difficult to find one who is accepting new patients. If you can't find a geriatrician, look for an internist or a family practice specialist who truly has an interest in and the skill to treat elderly patients. Talk with your friends, your parents' friends, and other medical professionals until you find a doctor with a good reputation and compassion

---

22 The doctor I found was on the Alzheimer's Association list and was lauded by the woman I spoke with as the best in the city, but I was told that she was no longer accepting new patients. Somehow, from an in-house list that I got at the Alzheimer's Association, I found her voice mail number. I called and left her a message, telling her all about Mom and pleading with her to accept Mom as a patient. And she did!

for the elderly, who understands the various different medical issues that face the patient with dementia.[23]

Tips

1. If you can, find a geriatrician! If you can't find a geriatrician, find an internist or family practice specialist who has both the interest and skill to treat geriatric patients with dementia.
2. Consider communicating with the doctors in writing, whether your parent has permitted it or not. It's important for the doctor to have as much information as he or she needs to treat your parent effectively.
3. Meet with your parent's doctor. The doctor almost always will be available to see you, even without your parent's permission. The information you give to the doctor—and your insights— can be invaluable to your parent's continued care. Parents don't always tell the whole story or the whole truth and can forget parts, gloss over important issues, or fail to recognize problems.
4. Learn enough about the language of dementia to be able to talk with the doctor. Search for a

---

23 For instance, one of the things that Mom's geriatrician told me was that I should call her if Mom ever had any sudden behavior change. Any infection or illness, in a person with dementia, even a minor infection, can cause serious problems with cognition. Look for a doctor who already knows that!

friend or a friend of a friend who can help you
learn or go to the Alzheimer's Association Web
site.

5. Be alert for sudden changes in behavior or men-
tal abilities in your parent. Know that any infection or illness in a person with dementia, even a
cold or an infected paper cut, can cause serious
behavior problems and cognitive changes. At any
sudden change, call the doctor!

6. If no one in the family lives in town or is available to assist your parent with doctor appointments, consider hiring a case manager or guard-
ian. The laws in different states vary; but these
professionals, who often have a master's degree
in social work or nursing, can take your parent
to doctors' appointments, monitor your parent's
well-being, attend care conferences at assisted
living or memory care residences, and assist with
many of the other responsibilities that an adult
child has for an aging parent with dementia.
Good case managers and guardians can be hard
to find. Begin your search at your local Alzheimer's Association, the Alzheimer's Association Web
site (www.alz.org) or the National Association of
Professional Geriatric Case Managers, Inc., Web
site (www.caremanager.org). Be sure to review
the credentials and carefully check references of
any applicant. They can be expensive: when you
do find one, case managers sometimes bill their
time at $75.00 to $125.00 per hour.

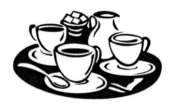

Chapter 6: Late Stage

Late-stage Alzheimer's is an exhausting stage. I remember—when Mom was in middle-stage Alzheimer's—looking at the people with late stage and thinking it would be so much easier when Mom reached that stage. At least there would be no endless arguments and tears. And it's true, there aren't. But there are still many challenges.

Communication is very difficult because there is less and less about which to communicate. There's no longer any traditional give-and-take to the conversation because Mom can't form words. Most of what she says is what they call "word salad"—bits and pieces of words—although she occasionally can form two or three consecutive words or get a look on her face that shows what she's thinking.

What seems to work best is to have a conversation as though she were participating, even though she's not: if she says anything at all, I respond to her as though she made an appropriate response. That way we can have, if not a conversation, the imitation of a conversation, and we can enjoy the comfort of the cadence of ordinary social interaction. This seems to work particularly well if there are three or four people talking, because then there are more folks to add to the conversation.

Poking gentle fun at other people can be particularly engaging. One Friday during lunch with Mom and another resident I told Mom that the chef must not know that the requirement that Catholics eat only fish on Fridays was eliminated during Vatican II in 1962, or else he would have served Rueben sandwiches that day rather than rubber fish and chips. The other resident at the table, Doreen,[24] laughed so hard I thought she was going to fall off her wheelchair.

I marvel at how Mom's methods of communication have changed. She never used to touch anyone, and she always hated to be touched. When she first moved to memory care, whenever people tried to hug her, she would angrily pull away or cry. Now that she is in late

---

24 Doreen is a wonderful lady who, at one time, spoke seven languages. Now, while she has very little language left, she is very alert and *always* laughs at my jokes. People who don't know Doreen are often put off by her, because if she doesn't like you she will simply pretend to be asleep. One of my favorite encounters with Doreen was one day when she appeared to be sleeping. I knew to ask, "Are you sleeping, Doreen?" She was mad that day, so she answered, "Yes, I am!"

stage, she seems to enjoy being touched or having her hand held. It was hard for me to learn to touch her after a lifetime of her living in her own little bubble, and me in mine.

But it was important to learn. One day I took my friend Yong, who is Korean and a hair designer out to see Mom. Mom had become extremely stressed during her last haircuts, and I thought it might be less stressful for her to have her hair cut in the memory care residence, rather than next door in the beauty salon. Plus, I thought that a less direct approach might be more successful, that it might be easier to get Mom's hair cut if she didn't really know she was getting a haircut. Yong has a Korean folk medicine background and is skilled at comforting with touch, but when she approached Mom I was very nervous for her and for Mom. However, Mom had changed; she enjoyed having Yong slowly rub lotion into her hands and arms, and even into her feet and legs. Yong was able to move from slowly massaging Mom's arms to stroking her hair and head and to cutting her hair. Mom offered no objection. It's hard for me to remember that I have to be changing as fast as Mom seems to in order to communicate with her.

Sometimes, the changes are totally unexpected to those who are uninitiated in the subtle ways of dementia. One morning I arrived to visit Mom to get a report that Mom was very agitated, so a caregiver was helping her change. When I asked what was wrong, assuming that she'd spilled something on herself, one of the caregivers said that Mom had arrived at the Village of No Stripes. I had no clue what she was talking about but learned that Alzheimer's patients often reach a stage where any stripe or discernable pattern in anything around them makes them very agitated. I learned later that this is because the patterns or stripes actually strobe—they move around because of the neurological changes happening in the residents' brains. Unfortunately, all her life Mom had been a big fan of paisley prints. Now, she can wear nothing with a paisley print on it. Solid colors are all she can wear. I also have learned that stripes and prints show up where I least expect them. One day I found that a helpful caregiver had covered Mom with a fluorescent-orange, plaid lap robe. The caregiver, new to dementia care, hadn't learned yet about the Village of No Stripes.

The other thing I've learned visiting Mom is that I never know when I walk in to the memory care residence what the benefit of the visit will be. Sometimes it isn't clear until I've left exactly why I was there or who I was there to visit. At first I would be frustrated when Mom was having a terrible day and I couldn't do anything for her; at other times, she would say hateful things to me or walk away. Relatives of other residents would tell me what a good conversation they'd had with Mom the week before, or how happy she had seemed sitting in the garden or planting flowers. I was jealous and wondered why I couldn't have the good times, why they got them when I visited so often. Then I began to realize that the visits aren't about me and sometimes may not even be about Mom. As I got to know the other residents, I began to see that sometimes I could brighten another resident's day. I, in turn, remember to tell their relatives about these good times. Relatives are all so happy to hear about any good time that it's important to share these good times frequently.

Finally I realized that, if Mom's being cranky, or having a bad day or, now in late stage, if she's asleep, that it's not a failed visit. Instead, it's an opportunity to spend some time with someone else. Once again, it's key to be flexible. Perhaps another resident could use some attention. I remember walking in one day, taking coffee to Mom, and saying to her, as she was sitting by Doreen, "Hey, Mom, let's have some coffee!" Doreen answered in a terribly excited manner, "Jan, how wonderful to see you. How did you get here?" This is the longest and most complete sentence I've ever heard Doreen say. I had absolutely no idea who Jan was, but I just couldn't leave her after such a response, so the three of us had a tea party. Mom was having a very quiet day, but Doreen was very verbal. The three of us managed to chat together for half an hour in what I think might have looked like normal conversation and, I suspect, felt a bit like that to Mom and Doreen. By the end, we were all exhausted but happy. I found out later that Jan is Doreen's daughter who died several years ago in an automobile accident.

Now, when I walk into the memory care residence where Mom lives, I try to be open about the reason that I'm there. The visit might be for Mom, but it might be for someone else. Sometimes it's for another resident or sometimes for a caregiver or med aide who needs to talk, who needs to hear what a good job she's doing even though she's exhausted and sad that a resident has died. Sometimes the lady at the front desk or the director needs a smile or a joke. Sometimes it's for me. Often, when I'm feeling forlorn or depressed, I'm intercepted by one of the staff and I feel better after talking with them or by a resident who needs a hug—but it's me who ends up feeling better.

Tips

1. Be flexible. Every day presents new changes and new challenges. Your parent may or may not need you—or be in the mood to see you—on any given day.
2. Recognize that every visit might not be for your parent. Some days you'll be there for someone else; but other people, on other days, will be there for your parent.
3. Share the good times. Get to know the families of other residents and pass along every positive interaction.
4. Be open to new forms of communication. The way that you communicate with your parent

will change: watch for the changes and learn to adapt.

5. Be alert for the Village of No Stripes.

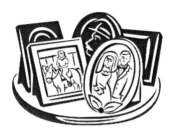

Chapter 7: How to Select a Memory Care Residence

Soon after the crisis, when Mom's husband had a stroke and she was diagnosed with Alzheimer's disease, I started looking at memory care residences. Mom did not yet need to live in memory care, but I knew she would one day. Even though I knew it was too early for her, I felt driven to check them out.

In retrospect, I think in part I was planning. I felt I had to know that there was a selection of satisfactory places where she could live. I knew very little about memory care residences, and I was a little concerned that it might be like signing my kids up for kindergarten: one friend once told me that if I didn't call several kindergartens to get on the waiting lists the moment I knew I was pregnant, my kids might not get in. Subconsciously, I needed to know that my caring for Mom, worrying day and night that she might wander off or hurt herself, was a stage that would someday end. I wanted to know that there were places she could go where she would be physically safe and relatively happy.

Each local Alzheimer's Association has a list of memory care residences in the area. Many are also listed in the telephone directory. I talked off the record with the staff of the clinic that diagnosed Mom and with Mom's doctor, as well. While many physicians are reluctant to recommend a residence, sometimes you can get a feeling for which ones you should avoid. I started with a long list and knew I needed a way to compare the places I looked at as well as a way to get information to my siblings without spending all day on the phone with them. So I created a checklist that I filled out at each residence and e-mailed that evening to my siblings. (See Appendix.)

While the checklist is helpful, I discovered what was most important was to be true to my instincts. It is important that every sense be on alert when considering a memory care residence. Look carefully to see if things are clean. Is the color scheme pleasing? Is it inviting without being agitating?[25] Are the caregivers caring for residents, or are they gathered at the end of the hallway chatting? Does the residence smell of sickness or urine? While directors of many

25 Remember the Village of No Stripes from Chapter 6. Does the staff know that prints can agitate memory care residents?

care residences will tell you that there's no way to avoid a smell, not all memory care residences smell bad. Find one that doesn't. What is the ratio of residents to caregivers? What's the caregiver turnover rate? Is there a nurse on duty or at least on call twenty-four hours a day, seven days a week? Are the services your parent will need available within the residence?[26]

Most importantly, watch the caregivers. Do the caregivers care about the residents? Do they *like* the residents? While caregivers have good days and bad days, as a general rule, if they don't like the residents, you don't want your family member to be there. Caregivers should receive training about caring for people with memory disorders; I believe that the ability to care for memory-disabled people is a gift, but proper training is also essential. The combination of compassion, patience, and authority that is needed to be a good caregiver is hard to learn, although some people seem born with these gifts. The good caregiver will have great communication skills, good intuition, and love for humanity.

---

26 Ultimately, it became impossible for me to take Mom out of her memory care residence. So, if a service that she needed wasn't available within the residence, I had to make special arrangements to get the service to her. While you may not initially think that a beauty salon is important, at some point your parent will need a haircut. It's much easier to have a hairdresser on the premises than to find one who will go to your parent.

For the first visit, I made an appointment with the community relations person at the residence. After I found a couple of memory care residences that I liked, I went back several times, at different times of the day and at least twice *without* an appointment. Find out what's going on when no one on staff at the memory care residence thinks anyone is going to be there. Ask for the names and phone numbers of people who have family members in the residence, and talk with them. If it is a good residence, family members will be excited to talk about it. Consider what activities the residence has for both residents and family members. Is there an Alzheimer's support group connected with the residence? Does the residence schedule family activities?

I found that having some idea about what memory care residences were available and where they were, and to have Mom signed up on the waiting lists of at least a couple, helped me feel less stressed. When the time came to move her to the memory care residence, I had some idea where to begin.

We knew it was time to move Mom when we began to wonder if she recognized us all the time and when we got the feeling that sometimes she didn't know where she was. We couldn't reliably find her in the apartment complex where she lived. The elevators in the seventeen-story facility where she was, in assisted living, began to malfunction frequently, and we were concerned about what would happen to Mom if there were a fire or other reason for evacuation: she would have no clue how to help herself.

Moving day was tough, but we got through it. The beauty of memory care is that the residents can relax. When Mom lived in assisted living, she used up a lot of energy worrying about the time of day, when the next meal was, and looking normal. She carried the same book around with her, day in and day out, and pretended to read, all the while looking for someone to talk to, to ask when dinner was. In memory care, no one needs to know when dinner is because there's always someone there to tell you when it's time to eat. When you think about the stress of everyday living, and the energy it takes to know when to do what, and how to do it, it's easier to appreciate the gift of memory care to someone whose brain can't process everyday cues anymore.

In a good memory care residence, the staff is trained to agree with residents whenever possible. One of my favorite examples of how important it is to agree is about a resident named Vance, who for years was an engineer in Hawaii. Periodically, Vance decides that he needs to go back to Hawaii to work on a project. Rather than try to convince him that he can't go, the staff encourages him to pack his bag and gets his airline ticket out for him.[27] They put it on top of his bag, and Vance always calls his daughter to say good-bye. (His daughter says that, unfortunately, he

_____

27 They actually have a mock airline ticket, with a flight number, in his name for him.

always calls at 2:00 AM!) She says, "Good-bye, Dad! Have a great time!" and Vance goes to bed. Then, the night staff unpacks the suitcase and puts the airline ticket away. By morning, he's forgotten. But he's had a great time planning to go. There have been no hard feelings that he can't go. The mood has been great, and no harm has been done.

Another good example of the difference living in memory care can make is a time when Mom refused to take her medication. She was extremely agitated, and no one had been able to help her calm down or convince her to take her medication (which was to calm her down). One of the caregivers, a gentleman with a lot of experience with the memory disabled, said he was certain he could convince her to take it. He approached her and handed her the pill and a paper cup of water. Mom threw the water from the cup in his face and screamed, "I hate you!" He got another cup of water and gave it to her and she threw it in his face, but she didn't say anything. He got a third cup of water and she threw it in his face and then giggled. He got a fourth cup of water and she took the pill. She'd spent her rage. I talked to him about it later, and he said, "She needed to take the pill. All I got was wet—and I know that I'll dry." Caregivers in assisted living or independent living would expect a resident to take medication without any fuss—and wouldn't understand how to defuse a situation like this one with Mom.

Be aware that, when you move your parent to memory care, he or she is moving into a living situation with other people who have dementia. Any item that your parent owns may be moved by another resident. While the staff tries to keep residents out of each other's rooms, there are some, particularly some of the women, who are known for "shopping" in every room. Many items will move around, so label anything of value. One morning, when I visited Mom, I was very surprised to find on the refrigerator in the common room a picture of myself, at age three, on a pony. Mom's new roommate had been shopping in Mom's side of their semiprivate room and thought it was such a cute picture that she'd put it on the refrigerator. So, label everything that you care about and perhaps, little by little, you can remove items from the room that you may want to protect.

Tips

1. Look at memory care residences long before you need them and get on a of couple waiting lists. Talk with the Alzheimer's Association, your parent's physician, and your friends—and your friends' friends—about good residences they may know.
2. Hold out for the residences that have no smell and where the caregivers genuinely care about the residents.

3. Label *everything* that you care about. Be aware that, even if you label an item, it still may get lost. Some suggest replacing valuable stones in jewelry. Others suggest not letting residents have any valuable jewelry.

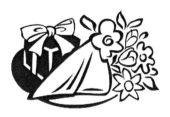

Chapter 8: The Care of Caregivers

The caregivers in the memory care residence are very important people. As the people who are with Mom twenty-four hours a day, albeit in eight-hour shifts, they have the highest impact on her life. If they're happy, then there's a greater likelihood that Mom is happy, and I'm happy. If they're unhappy, then unhappiness trickles down.

My experience is that, generally, caregivers are relationship people. Working in a memory care residence is a labor of love. Almost no one does it only for the money because the money isn't much. The residents in memory care work their way into the hearts of the caregivers. The relationships with the residents often provide the biggest incentives for the caregivers. Still, working in a memory care residence is extremely hard work, and the residents cannot always give back to the caregivers. I believe that part of my job as a family member is to make sure that the caregivers know how important they are to Mom and to me, that they get enough positive feedback and thanks for their hard work.

Turnover among the staff in memory care residences tends to be high, so one has to be alert for new faces. Even though I visit Mom frequently, I am surprised more often than I would like to be by a new face. I always introduce myself and try to establish a connection with a new caregiver the first time we meet. I learn their name and something about them and their families. As soon as there's a quiet moment (which may take several visits because memory care residences can be busy places), I tell new caregivers about Mom, so that she becomes an individual to them rather than just another demented, little old lady in a wheelchair.

Without becoming too involved in the day-to-day details, I try to stay in touch with how the working conditions are and whether they need anything that I might somehow be able to provide. By quietly observing and chatting with them, I try to keep up with what's going on in the residence and let them know, in a non-threatening way, that I'm aware of how things are going. I help out whenever I can, whether by bowling with the residents or bringing cookies or dancing during recreation time or painting the cinder-block wall in the garden so that the garden is a nicer place. I feed Mom whenever I'm there during a meal because I know it takes so much time. Meal times are good times to chat because the caregivers and residents generally are all together and seated. It's a good time to help out, because there are residents to feed, meals to serve, and residents who need assistance.

In many ways, all the people within the memory care residence—the caregivers and residents, the housekeeper and hairdresser, the activity and staff directors and the residents' family members alike—become extended family. I try to treat them that way, although it can be more taxing because to every visit, on top of seeing Mom, is added the cumulative stress of caring about the other residents, who are all getting a little worse, and the caregivers, who all have soap opera lives like the rest of us. Ultimately, though, it's more rewarding, and I feel better about the care Mom gets because I really know the people who are caring for her.

Tip

Make time to care about the caregivers. They have difficult jobs and deserve your respect, attention, and thanks.

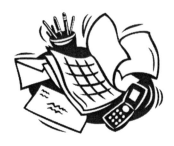

Chapter 9: Care of the Frontline Family Member

The histories and circumstances of every family are unique, but all too often there is one family member who carries the responsibility of caring for other family members. I have two siblings, each living at least several hours away from the city where Mom and I live. We are very fortunate that Mom can afford to pay for memory care, because none of us would be able to care for her in our homes. I am very grateful that one of my siblings handles Mom's financial matters. The rest of caring for Mom falls to me.

I do 95% of the visiting and 100% of everything else. I look for the lost lap blanket, go to the quarterly care conferences, wonder who the new director of the memory care residence will be, and make sure Mom has clothes to wear and toiletries. I oversee

Mom's heath; coordinate doctors, dentists, nurses, and beauticians; rearrange my schedule every week to accommodate some need that Mom has; and worry about the impact on Mom of three caregivers quitting. I routinely visit two or three times a week. On a good day, with no traffic, it takes me at least an hour and forty-five minutes, round trip, to visit Mom. Some particularly difficult weeks, when there's one problem after another, I am there nearly every day. I'm on call for Mom twenty-four hours a day, seven days a week, fifty-two weeks a year. I am the frontline family member.

I am not unique. There are many in my position. While in some ways it may be simpler to have one person in charge instead of a committee, the burden can be heavy. Some days we are overwhelmed and feel like we're alone to work out the problems. Some days we need shoring up. Some days we feel unappreciated because we're mired in our parent's health problems while our siblings live their lives without such cares.

To be fair, some out-of-town siblings say that the frontline family member doesn't want help or doesn't look like he or she needs any help. Oftentimes, the out-of-town siblings want to assist, have asked what they can do to help, and the frontline sibling has said nothing. Sometimes, the out-of-town siblings feel they shouldn't interfere, particularly if things appear to be going as well as they could. Some out-of-town siblings feel like the frontline sibling doesn't want them to interfere with the way the frontline family member cares for the parent. In all these cases, the job of the out-of-town family member becomes support for the frontline family member, not to actually care for the parent.

I have found from my discussions with my counterparts that, while every family is different, there are common themes to our challenges and frustrations. Sometimes it seems to those of us on the front lines that it would be easy to shore us up once in awhile. Here's a list for the out-of-town siblings, compiled from my discussions with other frontline family members, of some ways to help.

Tips

1. Say thank-you to the frontline family member at least once a month. Send a note or even an e-mail. It'll only take you five minutes.
2. Tell us we're doing a good job, because we rarely get much positive feedback.
3. Go overboard saying thank-you sometimes. Send flowers or some other appropriate token of appreciation.
4. Be open to being briefed and updated about your parent. Sound interested when the frontline family member calls.
5. Ask questions. Be interested in the issues that confront us as we care for your parent. Respond to e-mails.

6. Give us a vacation. Designate two weeks, once or twice a year, when the frontline family member can be off duty, in his or her own home. Someone else could visit each of those weeks and check in by phone another time.

7. If there are jobs you can do easily from the back lines, just as one of my siblings handles all the finances, do so! Everyone is good at something!

Chapter 10: Thanksgivings

I've been the Thanksgiving cook in our family for nearly twenty years. Each year, Mom would bring something, often a salad or the pies.

One Thanksgiving, over ten years ago, when I asked her to bring the creamed onions, she brought a big casserole dish of onions and canned potatoes floating in half and half. She couldn't figure out why the half and half hadn't thickened, even though when I asked she said she had just added the half and half straight from the carton, without making it into a cream sauce. She said it should thicken on its own. I also was puzzled because I'd never known her to use canned potatoes. At the time, this simply seemed strange. Now, I realize it was a clue.

For a couple years, she declined to drink wine because of her esophageal cancer, so I bought nonalcoholic wine for her. Then one year she forgot she had declined to drink wine and was offended that I served her nonalcoholic wine. One year she set the table backwards, with the forks on the right instead of the left, something I had never known her to do. Then she stared at the place setting, knowing something wasn't right but not sure what was wrong. Pretty soon I learned to save a simple task for Mom to do, because she would insist on helping but was unable to do anything to her own satisfaction, which made her mad.

A couple years before Mom went to live in memory care, her sister from Los Angeles, herself in the throes of early-stage Alzheimer's, came for Thanksgiving. She and Mom both wanted to help. I gave my aunt the job of putting the carrot sticks in the relish dish, which she did in about two seconds, and then she looked at Mom and said, "See! I helped already!" That made Mom mad, because she hadn't helped yet. They reminded me of two little girls, fighting in the kitchen—I think because they really were two little girls, fighting in the kitchen.

The year before we moved Mom to memory care, I asked her to put the cranberries on the table. She tried her hardest, but in the end she wasn't able to because she couldn't figure out how to move things already on the table to find a place for the cranberries.

The first two Thanksgivings that Mom was in memory care were extremely difficult. By the time of even her first Thanksgiving in memory care I was unable to take Mom out of the memory care residence. She wasn't sure who I was, which made me nervous to take her places; and she didn't understand how to sit in the car. The last few times she had been to my house, before she moved to memory care, she immediately had wanted to leave. Once she moved to memory care, she was very uncomfortable anyplace else.

A week or so before Thanksgiving Day, the residence where Mom lives stages a big Thanksgiving dinner for the families of residents. They set up long tables in the living room and invite family members to a traditional Thanksgiving dinner. While I know that some of the residents enjoy this meal, the addition of the long tables in the living room, the bustle to set the tables and serve the meal, and the dozens of extra people all create a calamity that makes Mom extremely agitated.

I attended the first Thanksgiving with misgivings, worried about what I was in for, for good reason. Mom had a lot of difficulty. I spent most of the dinner trying to calm her. The second was even worse: I had to move her halfway through the meal to a quieter room. I left both dinners feeling ill and totally anxious myself.

Before the third Thanksgiving dinner, I took time to reflect on the first two and tried to learn something from the bad experiences. I talked with the director, and we agreed that Mom did poorly during these festivities and that we would seat her and me in a separate room, with five of the other residents who also are made very anxious by changes in their surroundings and large groups of people. I told the director that I would feed Mom and Doreen but would not eat myself: I can't both eat and feed Mom. It's too complicated and stressful, and I don't enjoy it.

I arrived early and took Mom into the separate dining room. She was already quite agitated because of the process of table set-up and general hubbub of the morning. As she began to become anxious and cry, I could feel myself beginning to get stressed. Beatrice (another resident who hates these events) began to spell out loud (which is her reaction to stress), and I felt the whole event beginning to slide toward a great abyss. Wait, I thought, I have more experience than this. I've learned more than this. I needed to focus on creating a reassuring atmosphere.

So I started to talk, very softly, to Mom. We talked about how everything was going to be OK because everything was under control. I told her that everyone who was there was her friend and they were going to serve her a delicious dinner that she would love. I talked about my cat and my children and her high school friends, interspersed with assurances that everything would be fine. Pretty soon the entire table began to calm down. Beatrice stopped spelling. I fed Mom all her dinner and a piece of pumpkin pie. Doreen made castles out of her mashed potatoes and stuffing, painted the tablecloth with the whipping cream from her pie, and had a total blast. At the end of the meal, I stopped Beatrice from tipping herself out of her wheelchair in an attempt to pick up her final bite of pie, which she had dropped on the floor. "D-u-m-m," spelled Beatrice, sure she could have reached the pie if I hadn't stopped her. "No, she's wonderful," said Mom, clear as a bell. I got them each another piece of pumpkin pie.

And I was thankful.

Tip

No matter how bad things get, no matter how disabled your parent becomes, there will still be happy moments, often when you least expect them.

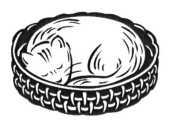

Epilogue
December, 2006

When I began this book, I thought Mom wouldn't survive until its conclusion. I thought that the final chapter would be an account of her funeral. But she continues to outlive every prediction. I am confident that there are happy moments in each of her days but equally confident that she would never have chosen to live this way.

There are great advances in the treatment of Alzheimer's disease reported nearly every day, with some talk even of a vaccine. But the specter of this horrible disease can loom heavy before the children of its victims. Personally, I've decided that, when I turn sixty, I will visit memory care residences until I find one I like, and then I will write two letters: one to my husband and children and one for them to give to me from myself in the event that they think I should move to a memory care residence. The one to my husband and children will tell them which memory care residence I have selected. The one that I write to myself will be an admonition to listen to my husband and children, a reminder to tell them how much I love them, and a stern instruction that it is time to move to memory care. I will update the letters when I turn seventy and again when I am eighty and again when I'm ninety.

Every day I tell my husband and children that I love them. I know that someday, if I'm unlucky,[28] Alzheimer's disease may invade my brain, and I will become my mother, unable, any longer, to string the words together.

The road my mother and I have traveled together has been long and hard, but we have had joyful and loving moments that I never would have anticipated, some that it took me too long to learn to see. I hope this book helps make the bad times easier and the good times even better for those who are just starting down this road.

---

28 There is a hereditary factor to Alzheimer's, but the experts say that you can have the gene and not get Alzheimer's or not have the gene and still get Alzheimer's.

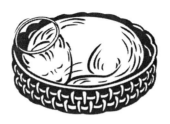

Epilogue to the Second Edition

June, 2010

I submitted the initial manuscript of <u>Unforgettable Journey</u> for publication in December, 2006. My mother died in early October, 2009: She lived over a thousand days after that final chapter.

By the time she died, she had been on hospice for nearly 57 months. She far outlasted every prediction. We never knew why she lived so long and we all said good-bye many times. Periodically she would have health crises that the doctors were sure would end her life, but she always survived. Finally, she simply stopped eating. She sat for three days in her wheel chair with a broad smile on her face that no one had ever seen before until she no longer had the strength to get out of bed. She died three days after that, peacefully, in her sleep. She had excellent medical care: she was never in pain and never afraid.

While the final thousand days were less eventful than the years before because Mom was so disabled, in many ways they were equally as grueling. Even as I began to speak to groups about <u>Unforgettable Journey</u> and the toll that Alzheimer's disease takes on families, I was still caught within its morass. While this gave me great "street credibility", I found myself listening to what I was saying to others and having to take my own advice. And I found that I never stopped learning, about Mom, about Alzheimer's and about myself.

The most important tip I now give to family members is to build two teams. No one can survive the emotional toll of having a family member with Alzheimer's without assistance. Build the first team for your parent. Find a good doctor for your parent; have some idea where your parent might be able to live; find a social worker/elder counselor who can assist with strategies and decisions about your parent. You might find one associated with your parent's doctor's office or on the staff of the residence where your parent lives, if your parent lives in a senior living residence.

Then turn an equally loving eye toward yourself and build a second team. Make sure that *you* have a good doctor. Find a good counselor: a social worker or a religious advisor or even both. You will need someone to talk to on this journey, someone to whom you can express your own emotions, sadness and disappointments and who will not throw them back in your face, ever. In addition, rally a close friend. Ask that friend to help keep an eye on you, to make sure that you take care of yourself. It is a great advantage to have someone you love and trust – ideally not a family member who is dealing with their own family issues – to watch over you.

Build your teams early on, well before you feel like you need them. You need to have your teams in place before the going gets really rough because when things get really bad you may not have the emotional fortitude to build your teams.

Too often at Alzheimer's conferences or online I see people who are overwrought: caring for a parent with Alzheimer's has stripped them of every inner resource and they are teetering on the verge of their own collapse. Usually a well-meaning social worker or psychologist tells them that they need to find a counselor, but by then they have no time or energy left for themselves at all, let alone to find a counselor. My heart breaks to hear a professional tell someone who is pushed beyond breaking that there is yet something else they need to do. I wonder if better advice wouldn't be this: Call your best friend. That may be all you are able to manage: call your best friend and cry. Then ask your best friend to make an appointment for you to see a counselor to help you put together a plan to recover yourself.

Once you have your teams, remember to use them. I wasn't able to make it alone; I'm not sure anyone can.

If your journey with your parent is long, know that your feelings may begin to change. Once someone is diagnosed with Alzheimer's, family members begin to grieve; each member in his or her own way, on his or her own timeline. Likewise, when the journey is very long, each family member reaches the point where he or she is ready for the parent to die. Very subtly we switch from looking for signs of life to looking for signs of impending death. We are ready for our parent to die for a hundred reasons: because the parent we know and love really died long ago; because we know our parent hates having end stage Alzheimer's; because we are exhausted by the demands of caring for a parent who is so disabled; because we emotionally need to move on and cannot as long as we must care for our parent; because we are desperate to return to the lives we had before our parent became so ill; because our own families – our spouses and children and maybe even our grandchildren – need and deserve our attention, too, and we need them as well. We don't talk much about it because most people don't understand, but know that you at some point on your journey you may begin to anticipate the end in a way you might not have expected at the start of the journey.

Prepare for a marathon, not a sprint. My journey with Mom was very, very long; most journeys are shorter but every journey is different. Think about having a plan that anticipates that you'll be there for the long haul. Have a contingency plan, or two, in case something happens to you.

In May, 2009, after caring for my mother for over eight years, I was diagnosed with breast cancer. I needed surgery, chemotherapy, and radiation treatments. I simply no longer could care for my mother and concentrate on my own health. I called my siblings and told them that I was done: somehow they had to figure out how to care for Mom from out of town. My brother picked up the responsibility, driving two hours each way several times a week, from where he lived, to manage Mom's care. I was very grateful.

I had never been seriously ill, although I had cared for disabled or ill family members (including my mother) for over 20 years. To be the one being cared for was an eye-opening experience for me.

Ten days after my first chemotherapy treatment my boys (then in the summers of their freshmen and sophomore years of college) dragged me to my oncologist. My husband was out of town on business for only a couple days when I got sicker than it seemed I should be. The doctor told us that I was very seriously ill, perhaps close to death, but I glared at my boys to tell them that I wouldn't go to the hospital. I was amazed when my boys cross-examined the doctor about his advice and then I saw the youngest, Andy, shake his head at his older brother Chet as if to say, "Go for it, bro," and Chet said to me, "Mom, you're not making any sense. You are making the wrong decision so Andy and I are going to make this decision for you. You're going to the hospital." A loud alarm went off in my head: **role reversal!** Wow, I thought, so this is what it feels like to have your kids take over. I was astonished at their courage. While I was unhappy to be going to the hospital, never have I been more proud as a parent. They were right: I wasn't making any sense. They watched for years as I made decisions for my mother and, when I was so sick that I was making bad decisions, they took over and made the right decisions. While I never expected to be in a situation so soon that prompted my kids to "roll reverse", I know that it was good practice for the future.

The other amazing part of having breast cancer was seeing how quickly the community rallied to support me. When I returned home after being told that I had breast cancer there was already a message from a social worker from the doctor's office asking if I needed any information or any help. Within an hour of my diagnosis, someone had called to help. Over the next weeks the American Cancer Society called; Susan G. Komen representatives called; people from my church called; my neighborhood rallied and cooked for my family for weeks (the boys were in heaven!); the world lined up to help. My doctors all communicated with each other and sent my records back and forth by email. Breast cancer, not so long ago something that no one would talk about, is out of the closet and society is fighting back with a vengeance.

How great it will be when we fight back like this against Alzheimer's! The medical community is beginning to move in this direction, but the infrastructure isn't there yet. And many families are still in the closet about Alzheimer's: they are afraid to ask for help. I have talked with hundreds of people since <u>Unforgettable Journey</u> was published. The comment that I've heard most often is, "Thank you for writing the book. I thought I was the only one." Families with a member with Alzheimer's still are afraid to reach out and ask for the services they need. And the service providers aren't reaching out to the families fast enough, in part because families are reluctant to admit to their needs.

Finally, when your parent dies, know that you may grieve very differently than other people do. When Mom died, I left a message for the son of her college roommate. Our families are only loosely in touch, the way family friends often are. I had seen him only a couple times in the previous twenty years, at the funerals of his parents. When he called me back he asked me why I sounded so happy. "Because I am happy," I told him, "She's finally free of the body that has held her hostage for so long", and explained that Mom had been entirely and completely disabled in every regard for the previous five years. Unfamiliar with Alzheimer's, he had a vision of Mom, pleasantly confused but functioning and living in an assisted living residence. People who haven't had the experience of having a family member die so slowly simply don't understand that we've been grieving for years, and we may well be entirely grieved-out.[29]

My journey with Mom is over. I can say with great gratitude that the bad memories of her furious and hateful outbursts caused by the Alzheimer's disease have faded. Her anger, unhappiness and fear largely disappeared when she became so disabled that she was admitted to hospice and in some ways those last five years were much happier than the five before. Perhaps that is why she lived so long. My happy memories of her are much more resilient than the bad ones, and I treasure them. I am confident that Mom is in a much happier place, brain entirely intact, able to read and dance and eat her oatmeal raisin cookies once again.

That is how I choose to remember her.

TIPS

1. Build two teams, one to support your parent and another to support only you.
2. Use your teams!

---

29 When President Ronald Reagan, an Alzheimer's victim, died in June, 2004, I found I couldn't watch any of the memorial services. Mom had been on hospice for 18 months by then, and I knew that at some level his wife must be full of relief. I didn't have the fortitude to watch her have to continue, again, in full public view, mourn a man that I knew she had been mourning for years.

3. Have an auxiliary plan: you may need an extended time off. Find someone who can step in if you need them to.
4. Know that you may grieve differently than anyone else and that this is okay.
5. Know that every Alzheimer's journey will end, even if some days it seems like it won't.

Eulogy for Phyllis

We are here today to celebrate: to celebrate our mother's life and her extraordinary achievements; to celebrate her amazing will to live and the tenacity and ferociousness with which she fought Alzheimer's disease; and to celebrate that she decided, in her own good time, to leave the body and mind that had become her prison, and move on to heaven.

Our mother was born in 1926 in Los Angeles, the eldest of two daughters of an orthopedic surgeon and a nurse. She attended public elementary school and Marlborough High School, which she loved and where she made several life-long friends and won all kinds of awards for her scholarship and her athletic abilities. Afterwards she went on to Stanford University for three years of undergraduate training before entering Stanford Law School. In 1950, she graduated from Stanford Law School, one of three women in her class, one class behind William Rehnquist and ahead of Sandra Dey O'Connor.

She married our father, a classmate at Stanford Law School, at Christmas time during their last year of law school and moved north to Portland after graduation. Mom passed the Oregon State Bar and worked as a title examiner (the early fifties were unkind to women lawyers) until she had the first of three children when she stopped working outside the home. I came along two years later, and my sister nearly three years after that.

As we grew, Mom became very involved in volunteer work as a member of the Portland Junior League. Membership in the Junior League came with a high volunteer hour commitment to various local endeavors, which she enjoyed very much. Eventually she became treasurer, and then president of "The League", as she called it. Every Thursday night she took modern dance classes with a very closely-knit group of women and later even taught modern dance at Christie School on the campus of Marylhurst College. A sometime golfer, she was happier playing tennis and enjoyed occasional roles as a member of Kay Lee's Playbox Players, a children's improvisational theatre troupe. The witch in *Hansel and Gretel* was her favorite role, with the grandmother in *Little Red Riding Hood* a close second. She read voraciously all of the time: Mysteries were her first choice. She always had at least one cat, often two. An excellent bridge player, for nearly forty years she was a member of a bridge club that stopped playing bridge after twenty years because there were so many other interesting things to talk about. Mom tolerated our family car camping trips (although they weren't her first choice) and even gamely suffered through one back packing trip, but most liked the family vacations to a guest ranch in Canada where she could ride horses. My brother and his wife just returned from a trip to the very same guest ranch.

In the early 1970s, when we were all teenagers, she and our father divorced. Mom brushed off her resume with aplomb and went to work as the founding director of the Volunteer Bureau, a United Way agency that matches up people who want to volunteer with non-profits that need volunteers. Mom loved working because she loved the people she worked with and all the interesting people she met. Four years after her divorce, on her birthday a friend introduced Mom to a friend of his from Rotary. Her friend photocopied his friend's page from the Rotary directory, folded the page into an origami boat and wrote across the hull "This guy will really rock your boat!" Indeed he did and they were married one year later to the day, on her 50th birthday. They were married for 31 years until her husband died in February of 2007. Together they enjoyed frequent trips to England and Mexico and were active members of their church, Moreland Presbyterian.

At the age of sixty-five, having won dozens of awards during her nearly twenty year career, Mom retired and began volunteering again in earnest for her church and the Citizen Review Board. For many years she was recording secretary for a book club as she once again had time to read several books a week. Although her Thursday night dance class ended in the 1970s, she regularly walked several miles a day through Eastmoreland, where she lived.

In 1995, Mom was diagnosed with esophageal cancer and told she had about a year to live. I don't think she heard the doctor. Mom simply beat esophageal cancer.

In September, 2001 Mom was diagnosed with middle-stage Alzheimer's disease. The doctor who diagnosed her disease marveled at Mom's determination and ability to cope without formal assistance for so long. She simply willed herself to keep going, always declining to ask for help and, frankly, declining the help that was offered, anyway. At every stage she fought the disease she hated, earning the admiration and affection of all who knew her in the process. Even at her most disabled, when she could no longer speak, she would tell us, with her body language and facial expressions, what she liked and disliked. For instance, she hated being weighed. She still loved vegetables, even pureed, but not so much the meat. Oatmeal for breakfast was still her favorite meal. She delighted in whipping cream and ice cream. And she never lost her life-long abhorrence for accordion music! Two weeks ago, she stopped eating. That day, and for two days after that, she sat in her wheelchair, her color was wonderful and she smiled a broad grin that no one had ever seen before.

The next day she was too weak to get out of bed and two days later she simply stopped breathing. She was never in pain and never anxious.

The last eight years of Mom's life were her ultimate struggle. One of the horrors of Alzheimer's is its ability to isolate its victims and their families. But Mom was never isolated. So, on her behalf, I thank her long-time friend, Ethelyn, who visited Mom until the very end. Mom had the very best doctors: Thank you, Dr. Marian Hodges, her geriatrician, who always returned my phone calls. Thank you to my dear friend Dr. Shirin Sukumar (also a geriatrician) for your extraordinary friendship and patience with my endless questions. Mom was well cared for. Thank you to 6 ½ years of nurses, med-aids and caregivers who brought happiness to each of her days, many of whom are here today: Thank you Sandy, Tedi, Daylene, Nisha, Lulan, Linda, Starla, Andrea, Crystal and many others. Thank you Sister Rita, a retired nurse and hospital executive director, now a hospice volunteer, who visited Mom twice a week for many years. My personal thanks to Betty Trowbridge, John and Sylvia Dilworth and the Prayer Team at this church who have prayed me through the long years of my mother's illness. Thank you to my husband and sons, who have abided patiently with me. Thank you especially to my brother, who has managed Mom's finances for many years and then took over all of Mom's care when I was diagnosed with breast cancer in May of this year. He hit the ground running and he did a fabulous job! Then you too, to my sister, who visited often even though she lives in the Seattle area.

Our mother was a brilliant woman who excelled academically at all levels of her education. Volunteering was her passion: she was committed to using her time and talents for the benefit of her community. She was a woman ahead of her time who, within the structure of the 50's and 60's, gave herself over to volunteer activities and then, in the 70's, launched by life-circumstance into the business community, built the Volunteer Bureau literally from the ground up into a successful organization, only to return to volunteering once she retired. True to her Scottish heritage – she was a Sutherland and we highlanders are very fierce and war-like – she never ceased to fight the Alzheimer's disease that was destroying her brain. Even at the very end, when Alzheimer's had five years before robbed her of her ability to speak, she would still, very rarely, fight through the tangles in her brain and say something. Six months ago, when her caregivers were getting her ready for bed, she began to slide out of her wheelchair. They telephoned me to say she had an "assisted fall". I don't know why I asked the med-aide if Mom said anything at the time because she so rarely spoke. The med-aide said, "Funny you should ask. She did. She called out – "Going-going-going!!"

Mom, although you are gone from this earth, you left on your terms, and, at long last, are off to a better place. And you will never be forgotten.

Anne P. Hill
October 2, 2010
Portland, Oregon

Appendix
Checklist for Evaluating Memory Care Residences

Name of residence:

Address:

Date:

Drive time/traffic:

Tour conducted by:

Phone number:

1. What is the ratio of caregivers to residents on each shift? What's the percentage of no-shows for shifts?
2. What's the turnover in caregivers?
3. What is the extent of training for caregivers?
4. Do caregivers have continuing training?

5.   Are caregivers licensed? Criminal background checks before employment and periodically thereafter?

6.   Size of small studio: Impression: Cost:
     Size of big studio: Impression: Cost:
     Size of one bedroom: Impression: Cost:
     Size of semi-private: Impression: Cost

7.   Availability?

8.   Waiting list?

9.   Levels of care and cost increase per level?
     a. Number of levels?
     b. How often evaluated?
     c. What's included? (bathing/dressing/eating/ walking assistance?)

10. Cost payable monthly? Quarterly? Discount for prepay?
     Price adjusted how often?

11. Month-to-month tenancy?   Long-term lease?

12. Buy-in?

13. Unit pricing?   Add-ons?

14. Number of residents?

15. Call buttons in room?

16. TV in room?   Cable?

17. What planned activities occurred last month? Are set for this week?

18. Movies some evenings?

19. Is there a secure garden for walking?

20. Exercise programs?

21. Are there supervised field trips?

22. Are there any special "buddy" programs for new residents to help them settle in?
23. How are meals served?
24. Meals available in room?
25. What is the frequency of housekeeping service?
26. Church service on Sundays?
27. Affiliation with religious group?
28. Beauty shop?
29. Laundry service?
30. Library?
31. Living room, sitting area?
32. How much time does a registered nurse spend on site?
33. Is there a doctor who is available for the residents, or do residents continue to see their own doctor?
34. How does the facility handle a medical emergency? Will you call us? When?
35. Who owns the facility?
    a. Is it publicly traded?
    b. Privately owned?
36. How long has it been in business? How long at this site? Other residences?
37. What's the biggest complaint that residents and/or their families have about this residence?
38. How many complaints were filed with the state each year? What's usually the nature of the complaint?
39. How old is this site?

40. Under what circumstances would a resident be asked to leave?
41. How many rooms are unoccupied? How often do you have vacancies?
42. Do you accept residents for the Alzheimer's facility from other than your own assisted living residence?
43. May residents receive end of life services, like hospice, at this residence? Do dying residents have to leave before death?

Other Impressions:
Think about:
Are people smiling?
What are the caregivers doing?
Is there any unpleasant smell?

LaVergne, TN USA
13 August 2010
193263LV00001B/2/P